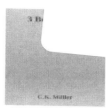

3 B...

C.K. Müller

3 BODY TYPES – A GUIDE TO THE (ECTOMORPH, ENDOMORPH, MESOMORPH) & AYURVEDA,

By: C.K. Miller

Table of Contents

Introduction

I decided to write this book, shortly after finishing A Manual for the Intermittent Faster. If you haven't read it yet, it is currently free for Kindle. If you did read A Manual for the Intermittent Faster, you would know that I got into Intermittent Fasting after seeing the results first hand with my wife Cheri. I have heard about the benefits of fasting for years, but, was very skeptical. I had been into bodybuilding and martial arts for almost 20 years and had heard of almost every fad diet out there. At first, that's what I thought Intermittent Fasting was. But, I soon realized that it was much more than that. It was in fact a way of life and one I still live today. But, I digress.

I'm sure we have all heard the cliché that not everyone's created equal. That statement applies to so many different variables. I mean I'm sure we all have one thing that we are really good at. You know, that one thing you seem to be able to do better than, or at, than everyone else you know? For some it may be a sport or other activity, and for others it may be mechanical, or technical. There is a saying I believe to be true;"we are all good at something."Even if that something isn't an admirable thing, because you do it well it makes you proud. So, with that said; before you start your training and nutrition regimen, it's a good idea to figure out your body type. All together there are (3) three basic types. Knowing which one of these three basic body types you're closest to will help you better tailor your diet and exercise plan. So you can set realistic, attainable goals that pave the way to your success.

CHAPTER 1 -THE 3 BASIC BODY TYPES

There is a lot of information on the web regarding these three body types and I recommend that everyone do further research on the body type category they fall in to. With that being said, all in all there are three basic human body types:

The Endomorph –distinguished by a prevalence of body fat.

The Mesomorph –distinguished by their developed muscular structure.

The Ectomorph –distinguished by a lack of much fat or muscle tissue.

So, what you have to do is ask yourself; when you look at your bare body in the mirror, which do you see? Because unless you have been part of some secret government program where they modified your genetic makeup or you're some sort of genetic muscle mutant, your body will fall into one of the three typical body shapes.

This idea that human body types are genetically predisposition into one of three categories is nothing new by all means. But, if this all seems like a revolutionary breakthrough, Plato mentions it in The Republic, which was written around 380 BC, and 19th-century philosopher Friedrich Nietzsche referred to the idea in "The Antichrist" years before the American psychologist William Sheldon popularized three broad categories of body in the 1940s. Since Sheldon's conclusions were published it has become widely recognized that most people fall into one of those three body types. In this Chapter we will go into detail about each one of those specific body types and how they affect both men and women.

However, with that said; although there are three distinct body types, it's important to be aware that most people share the characteristics of two of these body types. For some it may be a mix of mesomorph and endomorph, where you gain muscle quickly, but, also put on weight easily if you relax your diet. Then, of course there in that one that we all envy; the mesomorph. That guy, or girl in high school who seemed to excel at every sport they played, especially sports that require speed and explosiveness to excel in them. Who can strip fat rapidly from just a couple workouts, the Adonis or Aphrodite, the star athlete

Ayurvedic medicine has evolved from five thousand-year-old Sanskrit teachings, where body types and their associated personalities were defined as Vata, Pitta, and Kapha. It was Sheldon who introduced his theory of Somotypes back in the 1940's. His theory concluded that there are three body types and each body type has a specific personality associated with it. The theories that Sheldon presented have become a central theme running through literature and research with respect to weight loss, exercise, and bodybuilding. The body type system that Sheldon introduced to characterize the human body are the ectomorphic, mesomorphic, or endomorphic body types.

Not every human will fit exactly into one of these categories but contains characteristics of each. Although one is usually predominant over the others. In order to determine your body type, you need to look back at your adolescent years to determine which category your body type you possessed before changes due to age and lifestyle transformed you into what you are today. So, in essence genes do play a big role in it.

CHAPTER – 2 THE ECTOMORPH

This is typically a skinny person male, or female. You know that guy or girl that can eat and eat, and eat some more, and never seem to gain any weight? Everyone thinks they are a drug addict, but the reality is they just have a fast metabolism. Ectomorphs have a light build with small joints and lean muscle. Usually ectomorph's have long thin limbs with stringy muscles. Their shoulders tend to be thin with little width. The typical traits of an ectomorph are that of a delicate frame and bone structure. They have a fast metabolism and consist of mostly lean muscle mass. They usually have a flat chest with small shoulders. They find it hard to gain weight and usually look they have been on a seven day crystal meth binge. But, if they have always looked like that, chances are they are just an Ectomorph – not a tweeker.

That is because Ectomorphs often have a very hard time gaining weight. They tend to have a fast metabolism, which burns up calories very quickly. Ectomorph's need to ingest huge amounts of calories everyday in order to gain weight, so, workouts should be short and intense. Supplements are encouraged and recommended. Ectomorphs should eat before bed to prevent muscle catabolism during the night. Generally, ectomorphs can lose fat very easily which makes cutting back to lean muscle easier for them than an Endomorph.

Although the ectomorph body type is usually highly desired, one must keep in mind that they have problems of their own. Ectomorphs tend to lack shape because of their low muscle mass. Female ectomorphs are likely to have a flat chest and, wish they had more womanly curves. Male ectomorphs struggle to increase their muscle mass and may look malnourished. So, as you can see, they too, have to work hard to achieve their goals. Furthermore, some ectomorphs want and struggle to gain weight and muscle. The ectomorph has the body type that is most often seen in the pages of fashion magazines. They are slim boned, long limbed, and have very little body fat, but, also very little muscle.

Ectomorphs tend to have fragile, delicately built bodies and find it difficult to gain weight or add muscle. If you have an ectomorph body type; you have a thin, ruler body shape with narrow waists, hips, and shoulders. You may also be a combination shape like pear (ectomorph on top and endomorph/mesomorph on the bottom) or apple (endomorph/mesomorph on top and ectomorph on the bottom.

As an ectomorph body type, you're as delicate inside as you are outside. You're often introverted, artistic, private and thoughtful. Your skin may burn easily and you may suffer from extreme body temperatures. Your hair is often fine and grows quickly. The ectomorph can be easily spotted in any gym. They are often below the average weight for their height and have a skinny appearance. Ectomorphs tend to have very high metabolisms and often complain of relentless eating with little to no weight gain. The endomorphic body type is the complete opposite of an ectomorph. This individual will usually be larger in appearance with heavier body fat accumulation and little to no muscle definition. They find it hard to lose the weight even though they try many diets or workout regimens.

THE ECTOMORPH WORK OUT

Because Ectomorph's tend to burn calories almost as fast as they eat them, I would suggest keeping the cardio to a minimum. You are going to want to perform just enough to maintain general cardiovascular health. The reason for this is because you will burn so many calories while weight training. So, burning even more with cardio is NOT an efficient way to pack on any substantial lean muscle mass. The ectomorph looking to maintain cardiovascular fitness for general health and longevity should only do cardio at a moderate pace for 30 minutes three times per week. Any more than this is going to be detrimental to the goal of gaining weight. If you notice you STILL can't put/keep mass on, then restrict your cardio sessions to one day, it is OK to substitute 15 minutes of HIIT or circuit training into the routine as opposed to 30 minutes of moderate pace cardio. For strength training you will want to adhere to a push/pull routine with heavy compound movements and minimal isolation movements per each muscle group. You are going to want to follow a 3-day split so you can reduce the calories burned each week, lift heavy and recover between workouts. Rest days can be spread throughout the week, with at least one day of rest in between the last lifting day. I suggest doing abs at the end of each workout, performing two high-rep ab days and one low-rep ab day with weight. Remember that weighted ab routines can make your waist larger. The abdominal muscle is like any other muscle, in that weight training makes it grow expeditiously. So, be warned.

BEST WAYS FOR ECTOMORPH'S TO GAIN MASS

So, you've come to the conclusion that you are an ectomorph and you want to gain muscle mass. You are going to want to perform exercises with relatively high weight and low repetitions. Try to aim for the 8-12 rep range, that's where the most muscle hypertrophy (enlargement) takes place.

Also, you are going to want to perform exercises that integrate large muscle groups. So, do exercises that involve more than one joint. Dead lifts .are a prime example and great for overall for building muscle. They work your entire succeeding chain of muscles and are a great way to gain mass. Some other good exercises include bench presses, rows, lateral pull downs, dips, and squats; any compound exercises.

You want to eat foods that are high in protein. Make sure that you are taking in plenty of calories from rich, nutrient thick foods. Do not restrict your fat intake. Remember, if you aren't getting enough fat, then your body will produce less anabolic hormones that help tremendously with building muscle. Fats also lubricate the joints, which you will need from the heavy lifting.

Rest is one the most important and overlooked key elements to building lean muscle mass. Getting an adequate amount of sleep will not only give you more energy throughout the day, it will also allow your body to secrete more anabolic hormones. Try to get at least 8 hours of sleep a night. Light and sound play a big role in how well you sleep. The melatonin in our body activates in the dark. So, try making your room as dark as possible. Don't do too much cardio. Cardio is an important part of every fitness routine, but if you're trying to increase your size, then the cardio work will burn more calories. Try and keep the cardio to shorter, more intense bouts rather than long endurance type activities.

Although ectomorphs can sometimes be seen as skinny or frail, there are some advantages to having this body type. Every pound of muscle you gain will look larger and more defined than it would on someone with a larger frame. Having a fast metabolism can be very nice, allowing you to eat fairly large amounts of food without worrying about your caloric intake as much as someone else might have to. Ectomorphs excel in aerobic and endurance sports.

Alright, so now that you know who are ectomorphs and whether or not you fall into their category. So, now let's talk about diet plans for the ectomorph.

By now it should go without saying that for ectomorphs to gain muscle and put on weight, they will need to start eating more calories than they usually do. Unlike the popular belief, tracking calories is as important for ectomorphs as those on a weight-loss diet. So, how can you do it? Well, To begin with, calculate the total number of calories you consume each day. There are various apps out in the market that will help you with this. Once you know your gross calorie intake, calculate your daily calorie expenditure by using one of those apps. If values of both intake calories and expenditure are equal, then you are probably going to see almost no gains. So, the trick is to increase the intake calories by at least 250-350 each day, so, that by the end of the week you are likely to have put on at least half a pound of weight.

You are going to want to take a cue from the first principle, and remember that ectomorphs need to eat food all day long. Having said that, it's also important for ectomorphs to consider the calorie bulk of the food they are eating. Being an ectomorph, you may want to skip all the food items with low calorie density aka food items you need to consume in huge quantity to make considerable calorie gains. For instance, a small bowl of cooked oatmeal contains just about 100-120 calories but proves very effective in suppressing your hunger and making you feel full. Therefore, ectomorphs are suggested to avoid such foods and choose high calorie-dense foods like dried fruits, meat, fish and whey protein.

Eating three meals a day will not work at all. Once you are on an ectomorph diet, you will have to eat at least 6-8 meals each day and at frequent intervals. Out of these meals, have at least 3 major meals and 3 small meals or snacks. I would advise keeping breakfast, lunch, and dinner as main meals and adding healthy snacks to the routine between each of these meals. This way, not only you will able to keep energy levels high throughout the day but also ease the process of weight gain which may be a difficult task to accomplish.

So, now that we have discovered that we need to eat, eat and eat some more. It doesn't mean we can drive straight down to Popeye's and order 6 family buckets. Although that sounds great; if only life was that simple. We need to eat the right amount of macro-nutrients for the body to turn them into bulging muscles. There are three central macronutrient profiles we need to concern ourselves with.

,

Carbohydrates have been targeted by the media and, so called nutrition experts, as the route of all evil. However, this is not the case for an ectomorph. Carbohydrates are your best friend. You need to realize however, that not all carbohydrates are created equally.

Carbohydrates come under two main headings, fast and slow releasing carbohydrates, or simple and complex. Fast acting carbs, such as white rice, white bread, sweets, sugar, dextrose, etc. are broken down quickly by the body. Once you ingest these fast carbs your liver secretes a hormone called insulin. This spike in insulin is produced by your body for glucose metabolism. Put simply, it had to use these carbohydrates. If you're at rest and you have ingested glucose not needed by your body, it is stored as fat. However, taken at the right time, like say directly after your workout in liquid form, the insulin spike can fuel your muscles into an accelerated anabolic recovery phase. For an ectomorph this is good. For ectomorphs, building muscle is hard. They need to use every opportunity to create muscle and enhance recovery, so they may train again quicker.

Complex carbohydrates on the other hand, are harder for the body to breakdown. They give you a slower release of glucose when broken down and don't spike insulin. This slow release of carbohydrates is good for building muscle, as you are constantly supplying the body with the building blocks it needs, to stay in a muscle building, or anabolic stage. Unlike most of the world that seem to be running away from carbohydrates, you will need to consume large quantities in order to meet your required calorie intake. Remember, you are trying to bulk. You need to eat, eat, and then eat again. And when you're finished, eat some more. Stick to complex carbs such as brown rice, brown pasta, whole meal bagels, yams and sweet potatoes. Believe it or not sweet potatoes are probably the best.

Your exact intake of carbs will depend on your bodyweight but as a rule of thumb, take your bodyweight and eat between 2 and 2.5 grams of carbs per lb of bodyweight. Remember that carbohydrates contain 4 calories per gram.

You are going to want to also keep your body guessing. So, add in a day of super high carbohydrates just to trick your body so it doesn't get used to the amount of food you are ingesting. Tricking the body will keep it growing.

Protein is quite simply your most important macro-nutrient. Protein is the building block for body and is what muscles need to develop and build. So, it is very important for bodybuilders who are looking to add lean mass. You will need to stick to lean sources of protein if you want to create lean muscle. Yes, sure you can eat that whole sirloin steak, including the 10cm slab of fat attached to it, but don't complain if you gain a lot of fat and no muscle. Stick to lean protein sources. Turkey, chicken, fish, lean steak and mince, eggs and of course, protein shakes. Aim to cram down around 1.5g of protein per lbs of bodyweight.

Fats are often overlooked and for ectomorphs they are essential. Fats play a very important role in the body. They lubricate cells within the body, keep skin and hair soft and supple but most important for ectomorphs, they regulate testosterone levels. Without testosterone you might as well pack up and go home. Nobody ever built muscle without testosterone. Now that we know why they are important, what is the best way to go about getting them? Well, don't rush for the nearest bottle of oil. Know first that fats like carbohydrates are not created equal. Food high in saturated fat needs to be avoided at all costs as they clog arteries, increase cholesterol and increase your risk of heart related problems. The fats you are looking for are high in omega 3, omega 6, and omega 9. Excellent examples are oily fish, avocados, flaxseed oil, nuts or eggs. A mixture of all of these would be the best way to go about it.

It is also important to eat lots of fresh fruit and veg. In the UK the government recommends they eat 5 portions of fresh fruit or vegetables a day. Seeing as you will be eating more than the standard portion of 3 meals a day, I would recommend you try to double that. Fruits and vegetables are essentially carbohydrates so add them to your total. They also provide anti-oxidants to keep you fit and healthy.

CHAPTER – 3 THE ENDOMORPH BODY TYPE

People with the Endomorph body type are adept at storing fuel, with muscle and fat concentrated in the lower body. The endomorph is the hardest body type to have in terms of managing weight and general fitness. To get a more balanced physique, people with endomorph body types should focus more on developing their shoulders and stripping away excess fat from their lower body. A low- to medium-intensity cardio plan will help you tremendously in the shedding of fat, as will a 1,750-calorie-a-day diet that's high in fiber. If you have trouble shifting weight, the chances are you're an endomorph, characterized by a relatively high amount of stored fat, a wide waist and a large bone structure. Endomorphs tend to struggle with their weight, gaining weight easily and losing weight with difficulty. Female endomorphs are soft and curvaceous, and have a very feminine body shape. Male endomorphs have soft and round bodies, but when in shape tend to look more like mesomorphs. If you have trouble losing weight despite your best efforts, chances are you're an endomorph.

At one point in time; many, many years ago, you were admired and envied. When food was scarce, natural selection favored humans with fat-storing metabolisms. However times have changed. Now that sofas and milkshakes are readily available, those genes are hampering you. Experts have suggested heredity factors might account for as much as 70% of your body mass index (BMI). As an endomorph, you've probably struggled with weight problems your whole life – being chubby or even overweight. Maybe you were called "big boned" when you were a kid – you weren't overweight, but not slim either. But as you've got older it's become harder to keep the weight at bay.

The truth is that when it comes to body fat, endomorphs are on the back foot.

Paramount for endomorph's, there's no point in spending hours plodding away on a treadmill. The first thing endomorph's should start to lose weight is long, slow, steady-state cardiovascular work. Start doing more interval-based conditioning. Sprints and box jumps are great, but if you're heavy to the point of being worried about your joints, then exercises like the sled push are gentler but just as intense. If you're doing crunches, STOP. Focus more on cardio.Endomorphs are naturally strong and have good endurance and movement, and tend to do well in middle-distance activities. Endomorphs make great swimmers and also excel in sports requiring power and body weight force. Female endomorphs are represented in badminton, netball, martial arts, judo, field events (e.g. shot-put, discus, hammer throw) and tennis.

However, most endomorphs participating in sports, particularly at an elite level, are active, fit and lean. Therefore, they often don't look like endomorphs unless it aids their performance. Instead they appear less endomorphic and more ectomorphic and mesomorphic through nutritional and training programs.

Endomorphs lack the speed of mesomorphs and the endurance of ectomorphs, who excel in fast paced aerobic-type exercise and endurance sport respectively.

Endomorphs tend to gain weight easier than other body types. Endomorphs have a harder difficulty losing weight than any of the other body types. For an endomorph it is this vexing combination that has had led to many endomorphs fighting a losing battle against obesity.

Endomorphs tend to get poor results when following nonspecific diets that do not address and have not been adapted to their needs. What works for a friend, might not work for you. And emulating their diet or exercise regime that effectively transformed their body might do nothing for you. Endomorphs respond best to a diet and workout plan that takes their body type into thought.

Can an endomorph drop body fat and get lean? Absolutely. Endomorphs have incredible potential and a great ability to transform themselves, more so than any other body type. With a nutritional and exercise plan suited to your body type you can lose the fat and keep it off.

Intermittent Fasting

Intermittent Fasting may be best for those with the Endomorph body type. Since storing body fat for energy over long periods of time is a natural part of the Endomorph's genetic make-up, going long periods of time should not cause the same type of catabolism that Ectomorphs would encounter.

While much of the endomorph's focus should be on shedding fat through aerobic exercise, I am of the belief that weight-training is best because it carries on burning calories long after your final set. Also, the calories you ingest during the recovery period will help your muscles grow rather than fuelling your gut. Therefore, I recommend doing four days a week of hypertrophy training (heavy weight, low reps) alongside your cardio.

If you're an endomorph, you need an endomorph diet to minimize the bad gains and maximize the good ones.

Eliminating carbs entirely—otherwise known as a horrible diet—is brutal not only on the psyche, but also the body, hormonally, over time. Any diet that is too restrictive for too long is bound to fail, and carbs have a place in an athlete's daily regimen. One key to success is going to be understanding your macronutrients (macros) and knowing how to balance them. This is extremely important for the endomorph.

Again, the normal diet we are eating is terrible for the endo. Most of our calories are coming from carbohydrates. This spells disaster for the endomorph.

If you're seeking fat loss, you need to keep insulin at bay during inactive times of the day, meaning you carb cycle days (or even within days). Insulin is effective at driving carbs into muscle and liver tissue (good), but it's also equally good at directing carbs into fat tissue (bad).

To get the best of both worlds, skip the carbs at times farthest away from your workout or sports activities. If you sit in class or at work all day, replace carbs with healthy fats and keep your protein intake constant.

This means something like a three-egg omelet with spinach instead of a heavy carb-laden breakfast of pancakes and waffles.

One of the best things you can do for yourself is to start tracking all your food. Do it for a week to start and I guarantee you'll be amazed at what you see.

In my experience, most people greatly over or underestimate their caloric intake and therefore, have no idea what their BMR is. How can you expect to drop body fat when you don't have any idea how many calories you need? You can't. It ends up being a guessing game and most of you are guessing wrong.

But don't beat yourself up, this is an easy fix. Start by downloading one of the many apps that help you do this and start tracking today To find your BMR, input your age, weight, and height and you will get a number. You will then multiply this number (your BMR) by your activity level to determine how many calories your body requires to maintain your current weight. You can then either reduce that number by 10-20% for fat loss or increase it by 10-20% for weight gain.

As far as your specific macros, there is no one answer as everyone has different levels of sensitivities, but a good starting point would be something like:

30-35% carbs

30-35% protein

30-35% fat

This low carb number will be a challenge for many endomorphs since they are typically used to eating a very high carb diet. You can expect to have an energy crash for a week or two, but after that, you'll feel 10X better.

Your main focus is to keep protein levels high. While you're trying to lose weight and curb your appetite, it's important to choose foods that can fill you up without blowing up your caloric needs. That's why in nearly every meal—especially during a fat loss phase—should be non-starchy, high fibrous vegetables like spinach, kale and broccoli.

If you suspect you're carb sensitive or intolerant. Science is starting to reveal carb tolerance variations from one person to the next, and it all starts in your mouth. Salivary amylase is an enzyme in your saliva that starts the digestion of starches in carbohydrates. The gene that makes amylase, AMY1, varies in number from person to person. The more of it you have, the faster and more effectively you digest carbs.

Researchers compared the genes of 149 Swedish families that included siblings with a body mass index (BMI) differing by more than 10 kg/m2. The single biggest factor determining variations in BMI from one individual to the next was the volume of AMY1 in their saliva.

What's the solution for those with fewer copies of the gene? Be present at meal time, eat as slowly as possible and really take your time at each meal. Simple in theory, sure, but eating slowly gives your amylase more time to break down the carbs you're eating. This evens the playing field vs. people with more amylase who eat faster.

It takes a lot more effort for the body to digest protein than fats or carbs. In fact protein requires the greatest expenditure of energy, with estimates ranging as high as 30 percent. This means you will burn up to 30 percent of the calories in the protein you consume merely to digest it—plus, protein helps you preserve lean body mass. If you're a calorie deficit, you want to maintain as much LBM as possible—not only to look good, but also to perform at your best.

KEYS TO NUTRITION

Below are a few nutritional rules to live by:

Limit sugars, breads, pastas, cereals, crackers, and other heavy starches. Also remove white flour and byproducts.

Eat lots of fibrous vegetables.

Limit alcohol. They are empty calories and your body doesn't need them.

Aim to eat a lean protein every meal, preferably 25-35 grams. Not only is protein the most satiating macronutrient, it is critical for building the muscle you desperately need.

Eat fat. Many endomorphs make the mistake of severely limiting or trying to eliminate fat because they think it will make them fatter. Not the case at all. In fact, healthy fats like nuts and nut butter, oils, fish oils, avocados, are crucial to the fat burning process.

Take fish oil supplements if you don't eat enough fish. Fish oil has been shown to have a positive effect of many deadly diseases like coronary disease, Type 2 Diabetes, and high blood pressure, that are common among overweight and obese people, and as you know, many endomorphs fall into this category.

Insulin Issues

Insulin, which is a hormone that controls how your body absorbs sugar and uses it for energy production, becomes an issue when you have an intolerance or sensitivity to carbohydrates.

As an endomorph, your body just isn't as good at using insulin to reduce the sugar in your bloodstream, which is one reason why eating sugary foods and high glycemic Index (GI) starchy carbs is a bad idea.

Eating high fiber, low GI foods may be a good idea and can help to keep blood sugars stable. These include:

Whole grains like brown rice or quinoa.

Starches like oatmeal or sweet potatoes.

Fruits. Raspberries, strawberries, mangoes, apples, and bananas are best.

Vegetables, especially green vegetables. Spinach, artichokes, kale, broccoli, and beets are excellent choices.

Many endomorphs also tend to have a slight to moderate carbohydrate intolerance. What this means is that your body will react poorly to excess carb intake and likely store it as fat versus burning it for energy.

This means that keeping your cab intake low (30-35% of total calories) should be a good approach.

One caveat to the carb rule is that the endomorph should always eat carbs after a workout.

THE PALEO DIET

I am not a big believer in severely reducing or eliminating entire food groups, but there is something to be said for the success of the Paleo Diet.

Why I think it's a good idea to at least try it for 6 weeks or so is because it eliminates all the shit from your diet and as an endomorph, you NEED to remove it.

Basically your diet revolves around the following:

Lean meats

Fish and other seafood

Eggs

Fresh fruits and vegetables

Healthy fats like nuts, seeds, and oils

These are all healthy things and while I'm not recommending you do or do not go on the Paleo, it's definitely with looking into it further, especially if you are struggling with carb intake.

One of the main reasons endomorphs struggle with their weight more so than mesomorphs and/or ectomorphs, is that endomorphs are very sensitive to over-consumption of food. This means that the extra calories are likely to be stored as fat; resulting in a greater predisposition for fat storage. As an endomorph you will need to monitor your calorie intake very carefully.

The calorie excess we're taking about could simply be a chocolate bar a day too much. That's all. On average a chocolate treat such contains between 300 and 400 calories. Let's assume you consume 300 extra calories a day. That would work out at 2100 extra calories per week. This amounts to 2.6 lbs (1.2 kgs) of fat gain per month and a whopping 31 lbs (14 kgs) per year!

This may seem crazy. I mean it's just a chocolate bar, right?! But this is the actual reality for most of us and the reason we're gaining the extra weight and struggling with it so much. Who even remembers eating that tiny little piece of chocolate! While many of us wake up one morning and suddenly realize we're overweight, it doesn't actually happen overnight. And the difference between an ectomorph and other body types is that ectomorphs have the unique capacity to burn off extra calories – their bodies actually defend against weight gain. Other body types don't.

Now, that doesn't mean endomorphs will have to calorie count until the day they die. But for the first few months you do need to closely watch your diet until you have a firm sense of how and what to eat. And at regular periods you might want to do a spring clean/ inventory of where you diet's at. Looking over your diet for any bad habits that have crept in, and then to re-evaluate and reset your diet.

Remember when you veer of course it's often only by a few degrees (or a chocolate bar!). You want to catch it and get back on track early. Before you've strayed off too far, gained a lot of weight and become disillusioned, discouraged, and feel you have to start all over again.

ENDOMORPH DIET PLAN

As an Endomorph you will need to concentrate on burning huge amounts of fat. You have to increase your intake of fiber rich foods and natural foods. These foods help in reducing the calories in your body and enhance lean muscle mass. As an endomorph you really need to avoid junk and/or fried foods and replace them with healthy drinks and plenty of water. In fact, the more water you drink, the less water you retain. Thus, the more weight you lose. I would recommend that you drink at least 1 gallon of water a day, bare minimum. Also, you need to drink water. Not sports drinks, or vitamin enhanced water. Plain old filtered water. Limit your fat intake to around 20% of total caloric value.

The endomorph's diet should include carbohydrates like grains, fruits, oatmeal, brown rice, sweet potatoes etc., Take 5 to 6 meals a day which boosts up your metabolic behavior. Implementing such diet would really help endomorphs to gain a good shape and body.

PROS AND CONS OF ENDOMORPH BODY TYPE

I'm sure a lot of us think that there are no advantages to having an endomorph body type. That the endomorph is only characterized by fat storage around the mid sections of the body; however, the reality is there are quite a few positive aspects of this body type.

Advantages:

Like mesomorphs, endomorphs can gain muscle mass rapidly.
Endomorphs usually have high physical strength and athletic potential.
Individuals with endomorph body type are best suited for sports that require explosive strength like weight lifting, wrestling, mixed martial arts, etc. In fact, in the world of mixed martial arts, there have been many champions with the endomorph body type. Fedor Emelianenko and Cain Velasquez are the first 2 that come to mind. Both were heavyweight champions and many still consider Emelianenko to be the GOAT.

Disadvantages:

The endomorph body type has a slower metabolism that makes it difficult to shed the fat.
Although, endomorphs cannot be classified as "hard gainers", having a slow metabolism does means more attention needs to be put on keeping the fat away than building muscles.

CHAPTER – 3 THE MESOMORPH BODY TYPE

This will be short compared to the information I gave you about the Ectomorph and Endomorph body type. The reason being is they don't have to do much, because of their super genes. I'm sure just about everyone has a friend that falls into this category and you probably secretly envy them. In fact, they have supplements named after this body type, because it's so envied. The mesomorph from genetic predisposition has the body others long to have. They find it super easy to build muscle mass, and are generally proportionally built.

Mesomorphs have the ability to lose and gain weight easily, are able to build muscle quickly, and usually boast an upright posture. This body type tends to have a long torso and short limbs. Women with a mesomorph body type are strong and athletic. Mesomorphs excel in explosive sports—that is, sports calling for power and speed. The reason for this talent lies in the type of muscle mesomorphs possess. Mesomorphs have a higher percentage of fast-twitch fibers and will gain muscle mass more quickly than any other body type. Their genetic makeup suits power and strength. For training, focus on moderate endurance training, high-intensity interval training (HIIT), and plyometrics. You can add in Pilates or yoga to lengthen with strength.

To maximize body composition (lean-mass gain, body-fat loss) as a mesomorph, eat good quality fats with moderate carbohydrates and consider timing your protein and branched-chain amino acid intake. There is no need for a pre-training snack on non-training days. So, you can skip it and just have coffee or green tea in the afternoon. Eat your usual pre-dinner and evening snacks.

CHAPTER – 4 -AYURVEDA, THE THREE DOSHAS— VATA, PITTA, KAPHA

Since I've mentioned Ayurveda a few times already, I thought it would be best to give you all a little more insight.

Ayurveda is an ancient system of health care that has been practiced for thousands of years in India, Nepal and Sri Lanka. It has now become popular even in the western countries. Ayurveda is regarding healing and balancing the body, mind and spirit. It includes different physical and mental exercises such as Yoga. Ayurveda puts also great focus on diet. The central concept of Ayurvedic medicine is the three Doshas: Vata, Pitta and Kapha. Health exists when there is a balance between these three Doshas.

In many ways, the doshas—*vata*, *pitta*, and *kapha*—are considered to be the building blocks of the material world. All three of them can be found in everyone and everything, but in different proportions. They combine to create different climates, different foods, different species, and even different individuals within the same species. In fact, the particular ratio of vata, pitta, and kapha within each of us has a meaningful influence on our physical, mental, and emotional disposition.

For instance, a person with a predominantly Vata foundation will have physical and mental qualities that reflect the elemental qualities of Space and Air. This is why Vata types are usually quick thinking, thin, and excel in sports like running. A Pitta type, on the other hand, will have qualities reflective of Fire and Water, such as a fiery personality and oily skin. A Kapha type will typically have a solid bodily frame and calm temperament, reflecting the underlying elements of Earth and Water. While one dosha predominates in most individuals, a second dosha typically has a strong influence. This is often referred to as a dual-doshic.

As I stated earlier every person has all three Doshas within themselves, but one is more dominant. The same can be said for the Ectomorph, the Ednomorph, and the Mesomorph.

According to the Ayurvedic philosophy, different illnesses occur when there is an imbalance in the Doshas. To bring balance to the Doshas it is important to eat the right kind of foods and to do certain types of exercises depending on which Dosha is most dominant in you.

For example, if your Doshas are in perfect balance you will not have to worry about losing weight because your body will adapt naturally. You will not have the urge to eat excessively or unhealthy because you will automatically listen to your body. Your body will naturally prefer healthy food and this is important if you want to lose weight. According to the seers many health problems may also disappear when your Doshas are in perfect balance, including premenstrual syndrome (PMS).

FInding Balance

In Ayurveda, it is believed that the six tastes: sweet, sour, salty, pungent, bitter and astringent affect the balance in your body. In order to have a healthy and balanced body, each Dosha type (Vata, Pitta, Kapha) should include and exclude some of these six tastes in their diet. Furthermore, Ayurveda also considers if the food is oily, heavy, warm, dry, cold, or light, in order to balance the body.

According to Ayurveda, there are some general guidelines for all three Doshas that need to be considered. They are:

Don't eat cold food. You should not eat food directly from the fridge and you should not drink ice cold drinks.

Be present while eating

Don't eat snacks between meals

Chew your food properly

Besides a proper diet that suits your Dosha, it's also important to do certain physical and mental exercises. For example, a Vata person needs to relax their mind. They would also benefit from meditation and Yoga exercises, whereas a Pita person tends to be very competitive and would be better off with a more playful attitude when exercising. American football or other team sports are great for a Pitta person. A Kapha person needs to stay more physical active compared to the other Doshas, and would benefit from tougher sports that requires endurance, such as long distant running.

In Closing

If you would like to know more about Ayurveda, you should check out a yoga studio. In fact you should check out a yoga studio anyway. Yoga is great for the body as well as the mind. It also doesn't matter what age you are. You can start anytime.

Whether you are an Ectomorph, an Endomorph, or a Mesomorph, remember one thing. Time waits for no one. Even Mesomorphs can't eat what they want whenever they want and not pay any consequences for it. A good diet and exercise are the keys to longevity and a good overall quality of life.

The main thing is to always set goals. If you are an ectomorph, set a goal that you want to put on a certain amount of weight by a certain time. Say 10 pounds in 90 days. If you are an endomorph set a goal that you will lose a certain amount of weight by a certain date. Once you have set that goal increase it. When we set goals for ourselves it not only gives us ore structure – which leads to a better quality of life – it also gives us something to look forward to. When you have reached a goal, you are rewarded with the self-satisfaction that you accomplished something you set out to. This builds confidence and confidence carries a long way.

I'm sure you have heard the saying "we are all equal." Well, whoever first came up with that quote was an idiot. All one has to do is look around and see this statement is far from true. But, as human beings we should embrace our diversity. Although we may all be connected to this engine called life; there are many different parts to an engine. Take a snowflake for instance. Each one is different from the other, yet as we see them falling from the sky they all look the same.

Remember that without health life is not life; it is only a state of languor and suffering - an image of death. We often find reasons to not stay healthy and often those reasons just don't hold water. Saying, we don't have enough time, or we are too tired are just excuses we tell ourselves.

Make time. Be diligent, be persistent. Don't come up with excuses why you can't do anything, because persistence will beat resistance always in time. An excuse is only good for the person that is using it.

THE END

94774534R00024

Made in the USA
Lexington, KY
02 August 2018